Trip To The Lake

By
Jamie Stonebridge

ALSO BY JAMIE STONEBRIDGE

Trip To The Lake
A Day At The Park
A Visit To The Farm
A Day At The Beach

And more...

ISBN: 978-1-98023-160-8

amazon.com/author/jamiestonebridge

THANK YOU

It is people like you that keep reading alive. We can all live through books. Reading alone or with others is a wonderful thing.

I hope this book brings you joy and happiness.

You can help other readers discover this book by leaving a review on Amazon.

Special thanks to Rachel Horon for her time, patience, and listening ear. Without her, none of this would be possible.

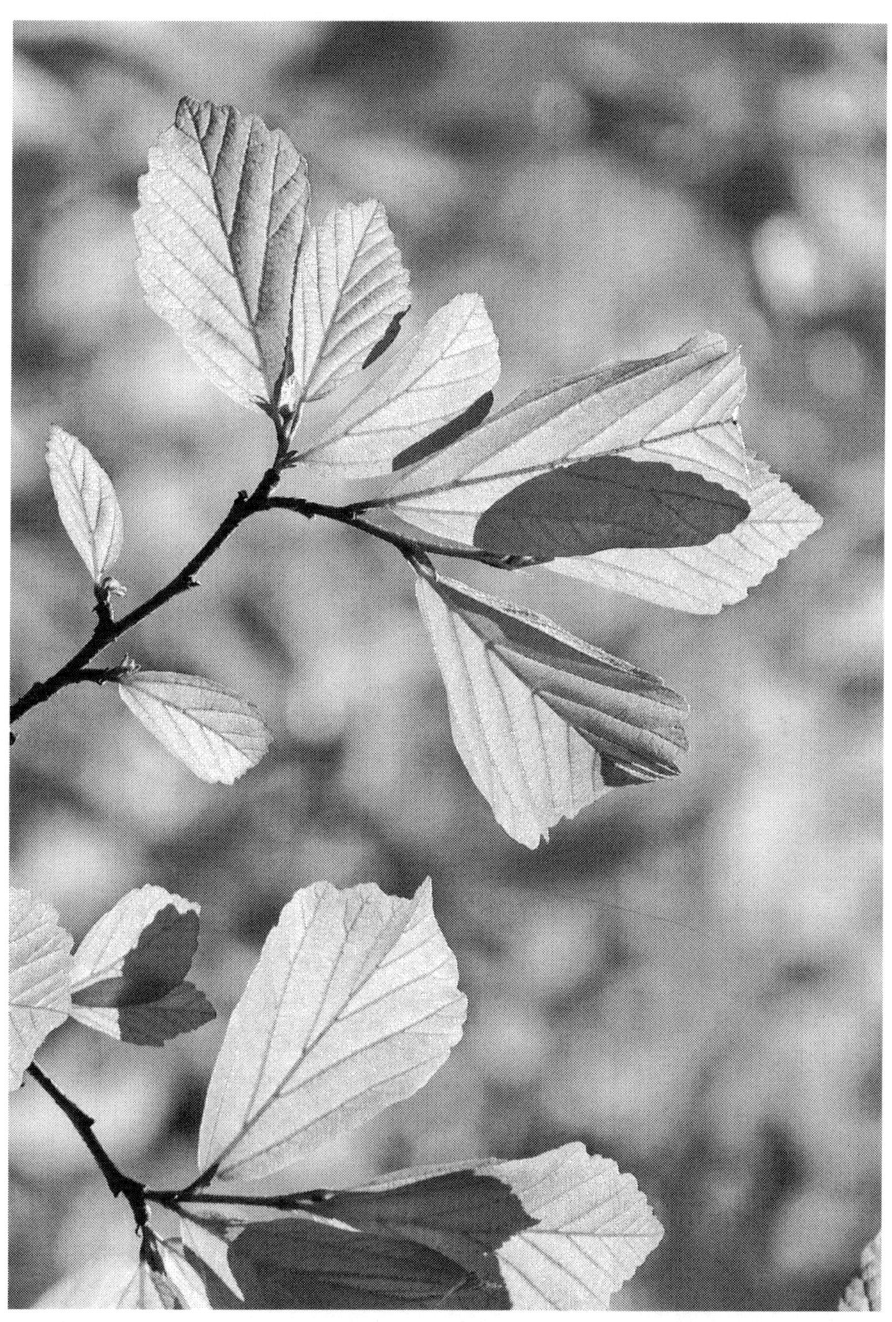

CHAPTER 1
Morning Breeze

WHEN I WOKE UP this morning, there was something in the air that was familiar, but fresh. I could see the treetops swaying in the breeze. There was a gentle roar as the breeze pushed through the open gap of my bedroom window. It was strong enough to make the white curtains rise and fall over and over. I could hear a chime ringing outside. I usually don't hear it that loudly, so the winds must be good today.

It was the breeze that made me want to get up for the morning. I was not tired anymore, so I got out of bed. It felt good to stretch from my fingers to my toes. There was something I wanted to do today, and the weather was very inviting.

I walked over to my dresser where my clothes were kept. There were some photographs in frames. I was in all of them and smiling. Most of the pictures were near water. I'm not as tanned as I used to be in those photos, but that is ok with me.

I put on a blue shirt and white pants. It was the same outfit as the one I wore in the largest picture on my dresser. I stood with a group of people in front of a big lake. The rainbow of colors of the sailboats behind us made me feel warm and happy inside when I looked at the photo.

Robert was already in the kitchen when I walked in for breakfast. The young man wore a green shirt with a collar and navy blue pants. He was one of the people in the photo.

"Good morning," he said when he saw me walk in. "How did you sleep?"

"Good," I answered. "My window was open a little. It let some fresh air in."

"Spring is here. It was a cold winter so I'm glad to see the sun some more."

I took a seat at the table where there were two placemats with red and white stripes. A blue mug and matching plate were set on each one.

"There is a nice wind over the lake today," he said. "The weatherman on TV said that the day is going to be a good one to spend outside. Want to go for a ride today?"

I was ready to go, but my stomach started grumbling. "I like that idea," I said. "First, I'm hungry."

Robert smiled. "Great. Your coffee is already on the table and your cereal is on its way."

Robert and I ate our breakfast together. He told me about his evening the night before. His daughter, Christy, played soccer at the park and made two goals. His twin sons, Michael and Jason, were too busy wrestling in the grass to watch the game. I enjoyed the stories he shared about his family. They always had something to do, and his kids always did something that was amusing. You have to have energy to keep up with children, especially three little ones.

I helped Robert by bringing my cereal bowl and spoon to the sink when I was done. While I finished my cup of coffee, I read the newspaper. Mostly I read the comics, but sometimes I read about the events in the community. It said that there would be a sailboat race tomorrow. That reminded me of the photo on my dresser. The weather today would be perfect for that kind of event, so I hoped it would stay that way.

"Did you see that there is going to be a boat race tomorrow, Robert?" I asked. I like to share information if I can find it. I may not be as busy as Robert with his family, but I like to share news with him whenever I can.

“Yes, they said there will be more people and boats there than in the past.” He was drying the dishes before he put them back on the kitchen shelf. “It will be more cloudy tomorrow than today, but the weather forecast is looking good for the race.”

“Will you be going with the family?” I asked.

“My wife, Nancy, does not have to work, so I think we will all be able to go. The boys want to see pirate ships, so I hope they won't be disappointed when it is just sailboats that are big enough for the lake.”

I laughed at the idea of seeing big ships with pirates and black flags with skulls on them floating on that lake in my photo. Kids really do have great imaginations.

Robert wiped his hands on a dishcloth before hanging it on the dish rack. “Ready to go?” he asked.

I got up from the table, grabbed my hat by the door, and followed the breeze that woke me that morning.

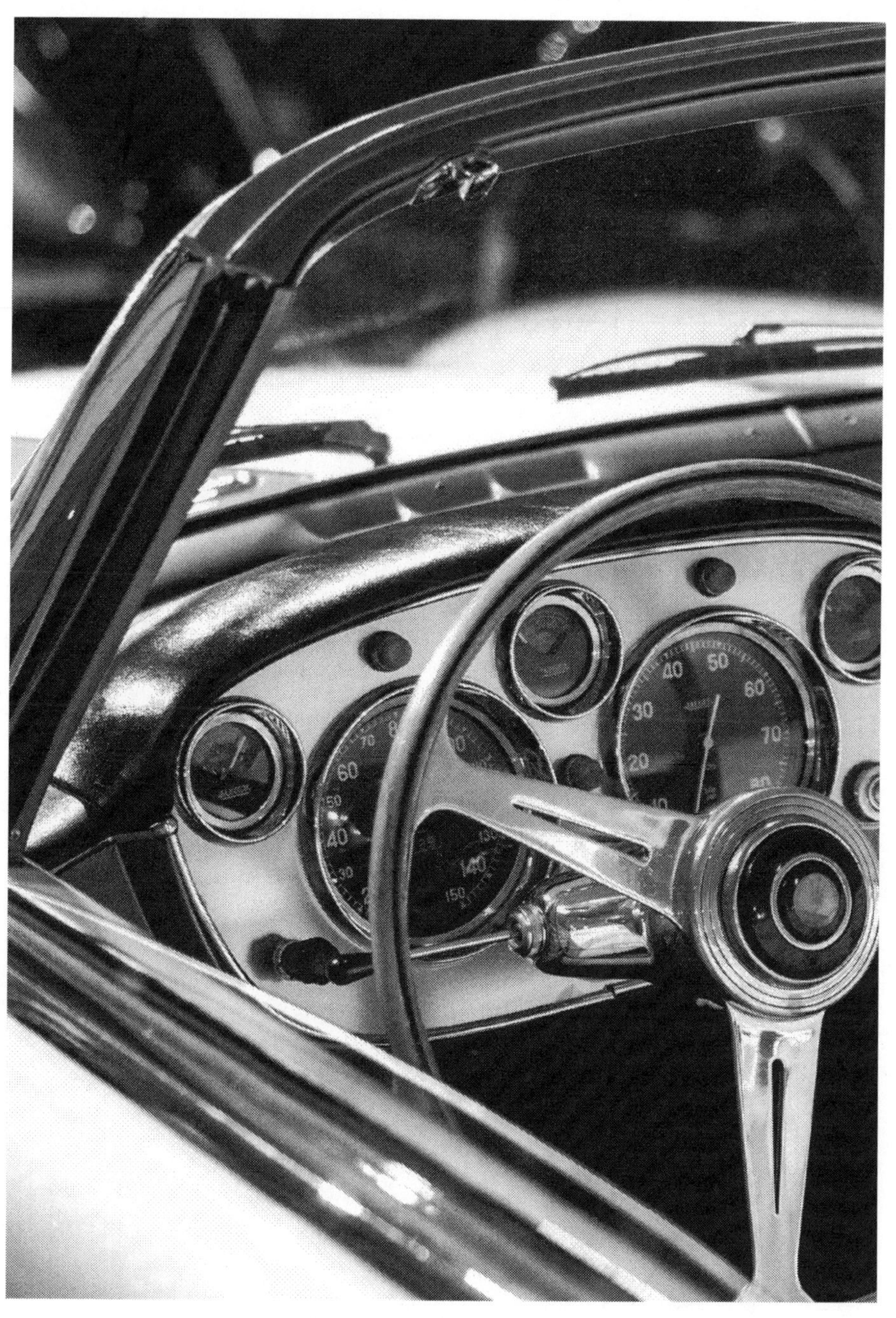
40 50
30 60
20 70
60
40
140
150

CHAPTER 2
Morning Drive

ROBERT WAS DRIVING this morning, which was fine by me. It can be fun to have control of the car and where it takes you. Today, I wanted to watch everything we passed. You miss the little things when you go so fast.

As we pulled out of my street, I waved to my neighbor. She was watering the daffodils near her mailbox. There were other neighbors outside who were also enjoying the spring weather.

We drove along Main Street. Some of the store owners were just opening their shops for the day. You could tell because they were still bringing out displays and placing them outside their doors. Some of the shoppers were ready to find bargains. Two ladies were standing outside the clothing store and pointing excitedly at something in the window.

I felt so happy on that drive. It wasn't cold, so we could drive with the windows down. My hat kept my hair from flying all around. My bare arm rested on the door frame and was warmed by the sun. Even Robert was enjoying himself. I could not see his eyes behind his sunglasses, but he was humming and tapping his steering wheel to the beat of the music. I was not familiar with the song, but it had a nice rhythm.

After a turn off of the main road, I could tell that we were getting closer to the lake. The path was more scenic, like some kind of park. The trees were taller and closer together. They blocked some of the sunlight which made the air cooler. Even the air was different. The breeze that woke me this morning had a stronger smell that tugged at my memory. Unlike the ocean with its salty smell, the lake's smell was fresh and clean like drinking water pumped right out of the ground.

There is something about the water that brings me joy. With each curve of the road, I got more excited about our trip. The trees started to thin out and the sky showed itself more and more. The robins and cardinals that sat in the branches of the trees in the park gave way to seagulls. It was interesting to see seagulls by a freshwater lake, but it was the place that they called home.

After two more curves and a hill, the blue lake sparkled into sight. By sparkled, I mean the little flashes of the sunlight off the gentle waves greeted everyone who came through the entrance. It was a lovely greeting and gave me hope for a great day on the water.

Robert pulled into a parking space close to the water. "It looks like a few other people had the same idea about visiting the lake today," he commented as he turned off the car engine. The parking lot was not crowded, but there were a number of early birds who wanted to be the first on the water today.

There were sailboats and kayaks already on the water, and even some people standing on boards with paddles. By the boat docks, there were some men and women checking their gear and their vessel. Their movement from place to place made it easy for me to see how eager they were to get their turn on the water.

Once we got out of the car, Robert locked the doors from his keychain. He pointed to a boardwalk at the edge of the parking lot.

"Let's walk along here to get to the docks," he said. "It will keep the sand out of our shoes."

I could appreciate that. It also looked sturdier than trying to balance in the shifty sand. We followed the boardwalk past the concession stand that was still closed for the season. There were signs and posters for the boat race the next day. Workers in safety vests were putting up flags and ropes along the boardwalk, probably to keep tomorrow's visitors off of the spring grass and new sprouts.

The beach itself was empty, mostly because it was a school day and a work day. The weekend and the race would bring more people out, but I'm sure the summer would bring just as big a crowd. Today, we had most of the beach to ourselves.

Robert led me closer to the docks and all of the different types of boats. There were motorboats and sailboats of all sizes, but I liked the sailboats the best. I love the idea of letting the wind take you where you need to be. When Robert stopped next to a white dinghy with polished wood trim, my heart started to race.

"Ready for another ride?" he asked me.

"Yes," I smiled brightly.

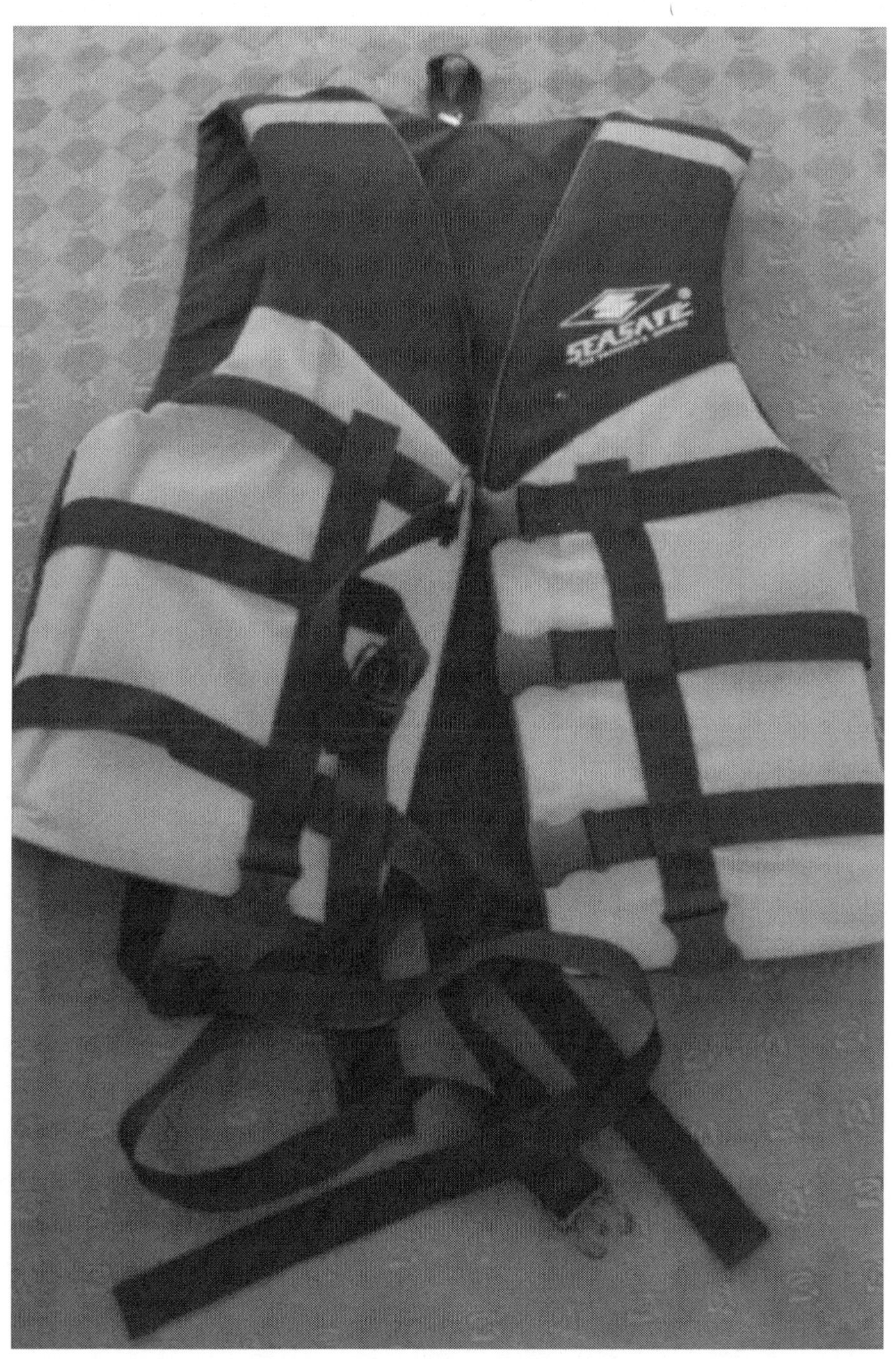
SEASAFE

CHAPTER 3
Setting Sail

WHILE ROBERT WENT through his pre-departure checklist, I leaned against the railing along the boardwalk. My eyes kept going further over the water to the sailboats drifting along with the wind. The familiar feeling that woke me this morning was definitely stronger here by the water. It was as if I knew this would be a perfect day for a boat ride.

Sailing is a social activity for those who like to be out on the water. As large as the lake was, you are still riding close to others. There are rules of the road and rules of the water. On the water, it is easier to see everyone else. In fact, those who were sailing close to the docks would wave to anyone they passed. I even waved a number of times to the smiling sailors.

"Alright," Robert said as he stepped out of the boat and onto the dock. "She looks seaworthy and dry. Just a few more things before we take off." He raised a neon green life jacket in front of me.

I wrinkled my nose. "I don't like that color," I said.

"True," Robert said, "but it is the best fit for you and it is approved by the Coast Guard." He smiled, "Besides, I think you will be looking at the water more than your life jacket."

He did have a point there. He helped me get my arms into the ugly green jacket and made sure the clasps closed securely. It almost hugged me in a way that made me feel comfortable and safe. I only looked down once, and after that, I forgot all about it.

I admit I needed a little help getting into the boat. Even though the water was somewhat calm, I had to hold on to the pile post on the dock and the mast on the boat.

Robert reminded me to put my foot as close to the middle of the boat as possible. I knew that, but my nerves made me a little slow. He stayed close until I could sit down and not wiggle so much. I wanted to wiggle because I was excited, but I didn't want to dance so much that we fell overboard.

As much as I wanted to help Robert get started, I sat back and enjoyed the sun on my skin while he set up the ropes and sails. It had been so cold this winter that the fresh air and sunshine felt as if they were recharging my battery.

I leaned my head back onto the headrest and closed my eyes for a moment to take it all in. The breeze was warm like a gentle touch. The seagulls were almost shouting “Mine! Mine!” on the sand, as if they had found a treasure that they did not want to share. But it was the smell of the water and the soft rocking motion of the boat on the water that calmed my excitement.

“And we're off!” I heard Robert announce. I opened my eyes. The ropes that had moored us to the pier were now inside the boat. The sails were raised and looking to catch the wind. A little flag at the top of the mast waved with enthusiasm as it showed Robert the wind's direction. Our boat eased out away from the pier at a slow and steady pace as Robert guided it with the rudder he used to steer. Once we cleared the shallow waters near the pier, we started picking up speed.

That breeze, that wonderful breeze, became stronger. My hat stayed on my head, but the hair peeking out wanted to dance in the gentle wind. Even the hair on my arms could not lay still.

We were catching up to some of the other boats on the water. I waved to the captains, young and old. When one wooden boat came by with the black Jolly Roger flag flying from the front bow, I shouted "Ahoy, matey!" I smiled as I thought about Robert's twins asking about pirate ships at tomorrow's boat race.

I noticed that most of the boats were circling the lake in a counterclockwise motion. From the dock to the far side, the boats were cruising along as if they could not catch enough wind. Once they reached a certain point, they turned and found the speed they needed. I could tell that Robert was heading in that same direction. I was ready for the next lap of our own race.

Sure enough, Robert turned the rudder and adjusted the sail. The noise of the canvas snapped as if the slack had been shaken out of it. With the new-found speed, we were racing with the big boats!

When he had the sail in place and the boat on the right path, he turned to me and smiled. “Are you ready to take the rudder, Captain?”

I had been waiting for this moment all morning. “Aye, sir!” I said, and he laughed.

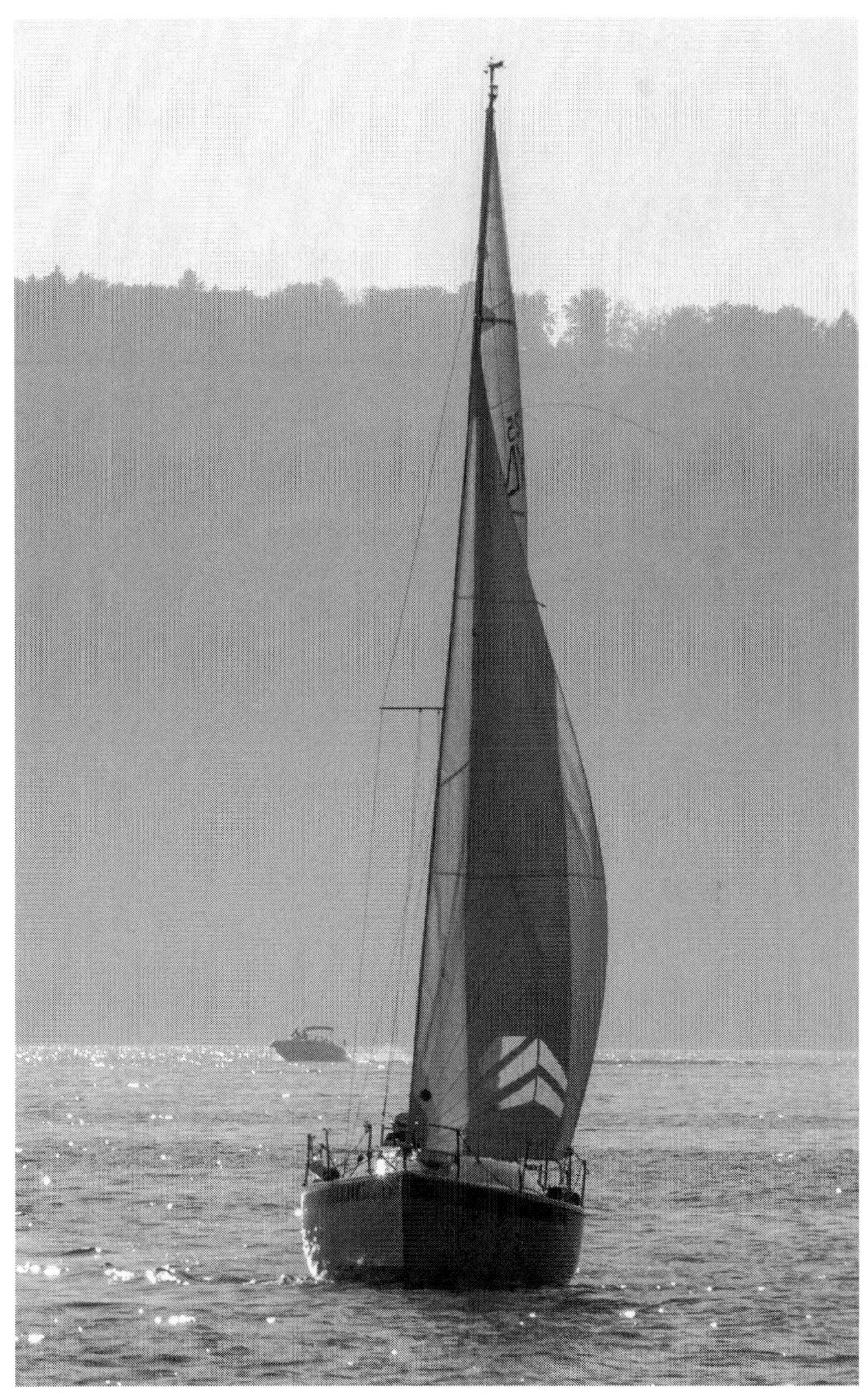

CHAPTER 4
A Good Captain

ROBERT TOLD ME that he would take care of the boom, or the pole that runs along the bottom of the mainsail. He was able to control the sail and the rudder by himself, but I just wanted to steer while we were out on open water.

Once I was comfortable in my position, my hand firmly took hold of the rudder handle. The boat was cutting through the water easily, but you could feel how much power the wind had over the boat. With one hand, you could change direction a little or a lot. If you were not careful, though, you could capsize the boat.

I did not want us to fall over into the water. Even though the day was warm, I knew the wind on our wet clothes and skin would make us feel too cold. The spray of water on my arms was cool enough.

I wanted to be a good captain of my own boat. Sailors can work on any part of a boat, but the captain is the one who everyone trusts to get them from one point to the other. I knew that Robert trusted me enough to do that. I looked over at him. Even though he was focused on the boom, he looked over at me and smiled back. We were having fun.

I was reminded that we were not alone on the water as another sailboat passed us on the right side. It had a larger sail than ours. It was white with a large yellow symbol of a sun printed on it. I waved to our water neighbors with my free hand. The captain was paying attention to the sail and rudder, but one of his passengers on the boat waved back.

The sun boat was going so fast that it seemed as if they were flying instead of sailing.

“They have good speed. I hope they do well in the race tomorrow,” Robert said. He kept watching the boat as it passed.

“Do you know them?” I asked.

“No, but I have seen that sail at other races

before. They must go to as many races as they can," he said.

We were almost at the other side of the lake when my hand on the rudder was getting tired. Robert took it from me and steered us around the lake with the other boats.

"Are you getting tired or do you want to go around the lake another time?" Robert asked me.

He knew I wanted to stay out there as long as possible. I was having a great day and did not feel ready to stop. "I think we can go around one more time," I smiled at Robert. "Unless you are tired."

He laughed at my joke and steered the boat past the pier where we had started. My excitement for spending more time on the water was as strong as the first time.

I was Robert's lookout as I watched for other boats coming close to us. I waved at the smaller boats we passed and looked for waves from the larger boats that passed us. I also looked for the sun boat to see how far they got across the lake. It looked as if they were going for another sail around the lake too.

Robert and I played a game as we tried to guess which boats were going to be in the race tomorrow. Some boats were easy to guess because they had symbols or pictures on their sails that were fancier than most of the plain white sails. I saw pictures of a star, a crab, and even a dolphin.

After the second time around the lake, I was

getting tired. The sun was higher in the sky and was making me warm. I was also getting hungry.

"Ready to stop for the day?" Robert asked me. "I am starting to get hungry."

Some days I think that Robert can read my mind. "That is a good idea," I told him.

Robert steered the boat toward the pier and found our spot. There were many open spots because so many people were out on the water that morning. When we got next to the pier, Robert took the ropes from inside the boat and wrapped them around the pile posts.

He helped me step out of the boat. "There is a bench under that tree," Robert pointed to a shady area near the beach. “You can wait there while I finish putting everything away.” He also handed me a water bottle. How did he know I was thirsty too?

“Aye aye, Captain!” I told him. The shade looked cool after our time in the sun. As I rested on the bench, the breeze found me again and cooled me even more. What a great day!

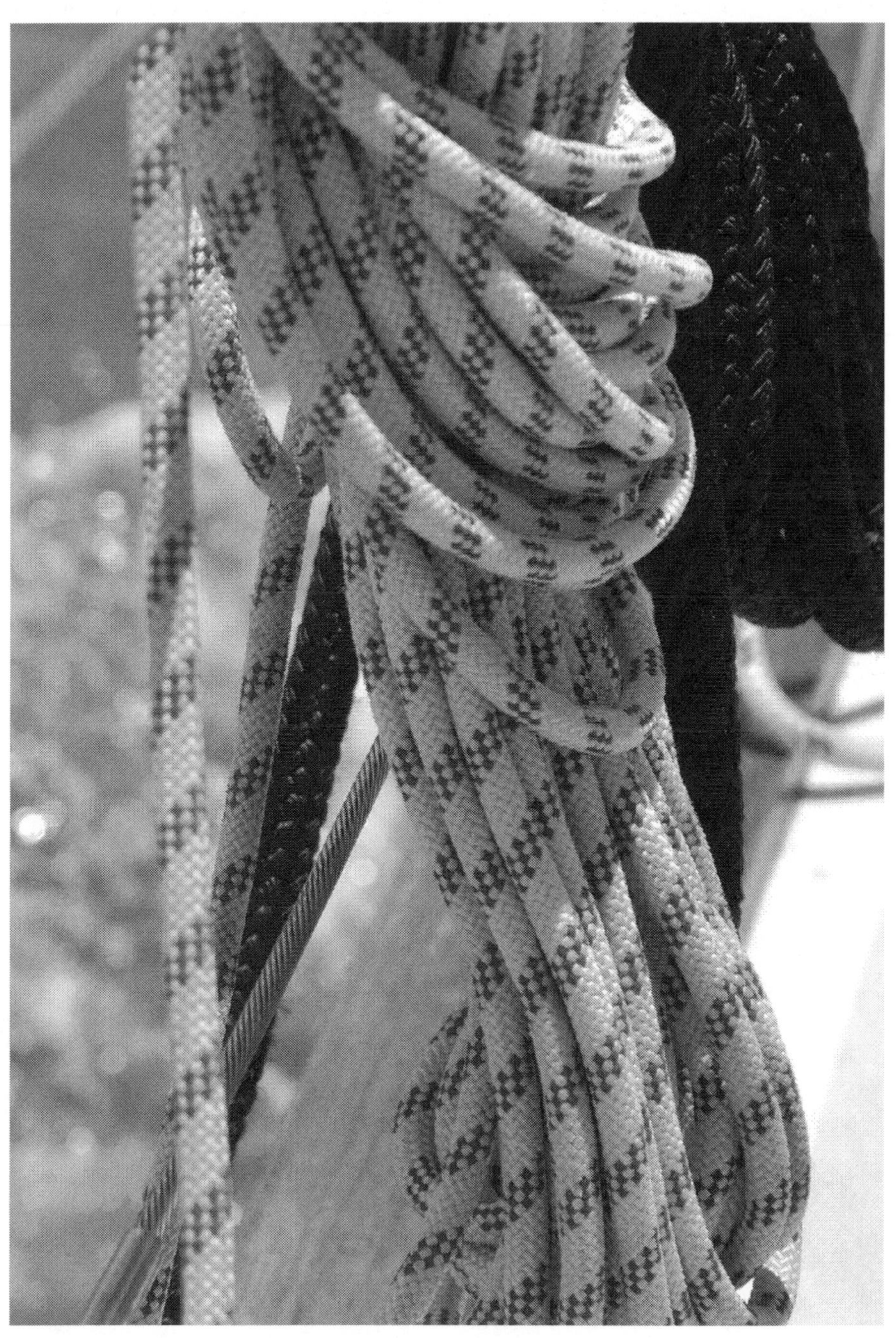

Chapter 5
Going Home

I watched Robert wrap rope into coils around his arm. The loops were big enough that the rope would not get into tangles or knots before he sailed again. I also watched the boats that were still out on the water. I looked for the different sails that we had seen before. All of the colors looked like a rainbow on the water. There was even a sail that had all of the colors of the rainbow on it!

Robert had a cooler in his hand when he came to sit down next to me. He had packed some sandwiches and more cold drinks. It was just enough to take care of my hunger.

As Robert and I sat on the bench, we would make a guess to see which boat would get to the other side first. Sometimes I would guess it was the boat with the biggest sail, but sometimes I was wrong. Sometimes I would guess it was the smallest boat because it would be so lightweight. I was wrong sometimes as well.

Before long, we got tired of our game. I was ready to go home. We cleaned up our lunch so that the seagulls would not eat it. We followed the boardwalk back to the parking lot. Even though there were not a lot of boats at the pier, there were a lot of cars in the parking lot.

Before we drove off, I looked back at the water and smiled. I loved our trip to the lake today.

The road took us back through the woods with all of the tall trees and shade.

“What did you like best today?” Robert asked me.
“I liked being the captain,” I said.
“I thought you would say that,” he smiled.

Did he read my mind again? No, he just knows me well.

“We did not see any pirate ships today,” I said.

Robert grinned. "The twins will not be happy about that. But I think they will like the boats anyway."

"Yes," I said. "They will like how fast the boats go."
"What do you think Christy will like?" he asked me.

"The sails," I told him. "She will follow all of those pictures over the lake. But I think she will like the dolphin the most."

"I think you are right," he agreed with me.

Robert turned onto the main road that took us back to Main Street. Since it was close to lunchtime, the restaurants had some of their tables outside. I saw people in clothes they would wear to work and some people who were just shopping for the day.

So many people were happy with their day, but I think I had the best day of all of them.

We got closer to my house. My neighbors were not outside like they had been this morning. They could be inside because the sun was warmer, or they may have been some of the people on Main Street. I did not need to see any of them today. I was just happy to be home.

Robert pulled his car into the driveway. When I got out, I went to my mailbox. There was a postcard from my dentist to remind me of my next appointment and a letter that looked like an advertisement. I was not interested in buying anything, so that one would go into my trash bin.

My house felt cooler than the outside. When I opened the door, the breeze came through the door and windows. After I put my mail away, I went to sit down in my comfortable chair. Robert emptied his cooler in the kitchen. When he came back, he opened his laptop computer at the desk and started typing something.

The tapping of his fingers on the keyboard and the softness of the cushions on my chair made me sleepy. I guess I was more tired than I had thought because my eyelids started closing.

For some reason, I felt as if I was on the water again. This time I was on a big wooden ship. There was not one sail on the mast, but many sails on three masts. I was holding a wheel with many handles. I must have been a captain steering a boat.

My ship was so big that I was passing all of the other ships near me. When I looked up at the top of the mast, there was a black flag with a skull and crossbones. Was I a pirate?!?

I woke up to find myself in my comfortable chair and Robert at the desk typing on his laptop computer. It was just a dream that had felt so real.

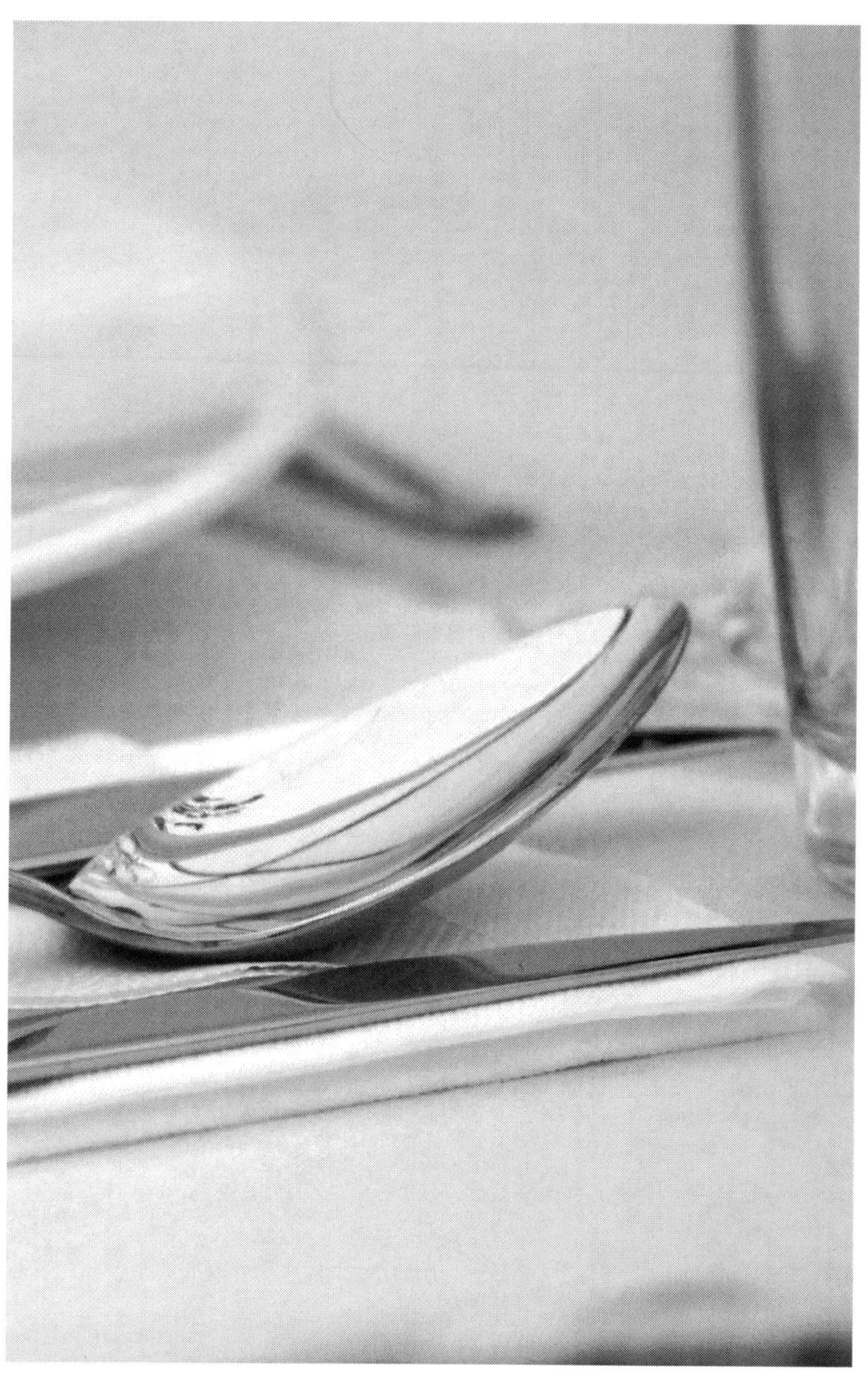

CHAPTER 6
Story Time

AROUND DINNER TIME, Nancy came over with her three kids. She also brought a pan of food. It was steaming as if it had come right out of the oven. It smelled good. I did not realize how hungry I was until I smelled all of its smells.

The twins, Michael and Jason, were trying to climb all over their dad, Robert. Christy walked over to my collection of seashells in the cabinet. I unlocked the glass door and let her pick up two. She found my magnifying glass and sat in my comfortable chair. She looked at the seashells closely, like a scientist in a laboratory.

While Nancy got the food ready to eat, I helped in the kitchen by getting out the knives, forks, and spoons. Robert got the plates and cups out of the cabinet. We worked very well together.

Nancy told us all to get ready to eat. I went to help Christy put away the two shells and we both washed our hands. Robert was helping Michael and Jason wash in the kitchen. After all hands were clean, we sat around the table.

The kids took turns telling us about their day at school. The boys were very excited about playing outside at school that day. They gave their report about a kickball game and how Michael kicked the ball over the fence. Christy was excited to talk about her perfect grade on her spelling test.

For dessert, everyone had a scoop of ice cream. I like vanilla with a little chocolate syrup, but the kids got colorful sprinkles over their scoops.

When everyone was done, Robert and Nancy washed dishes while the kids and I went outside onto the patio.

Christy was trying to solve a colorful magic cube. She was turning it in different directions trying to get the six colors on their own side. The boys were playing tag in the grass. After about five minutes, I called them over. “Do you want to hear a story?” I asked.

They ran over to get close enough to hear. When they had found stools to sit on, I started on a story that was like my dream from my nap that afternoon.

“Once upon a time,” I started, “there was a pirate captain named Captain Grayhair.” The twins giggled as they thought of a gray-haired pirate. “Captain Grayhair was the best pirate to sail the seven seas on the ship called ... The Salty Dog!”

“What are the names of the seven seas?” one of the twins asked. I could not tell if it was Michael or Jason because they looked so much alike.

"Red, Orange, Yellow, Green, Blue, Indigo, and Violet," I said with a smile on my face. Then I continued the story. "One day, Captain Grayhair was sailing when another ship tried to pass. It was Captain Sunnyside, the fastest pirate on fresh water."

"I thought seas were salt water," Christy asked. She had her magic cube on her lap and was listening to my story.

Robert and Nancy walked onto the patio to join the story too. "Some seas are like big lakes," Robert said. "But you are right that most seas are salt water."

I continued with my story. "Captain Sunnyside told Captain Grayhair that he wanted to race The Salty Dog. Captain Grayhair was proud of the crew working on

The Salty Dog. The captain said yes to the challenge."

"With the help of the crew of two twin boys and a smart little girl, Captain Grayhair passed Captain Sunnyside's sails with the golden sun on it."

The three kids cheered while Michael and Jason made pirate calls like "Arr matey!"

"And do you know why they were able to win against the fastest pirate on fresh water?" I asked. The kids called out so many guesses that I could not hear them all so I answered for them. "Because the best crew on The Salty Dog were smaller than the big crew on the other ship. The ship was lighter, and that helped it go faster."

“Is that true?” Christy asked. She also looked at her mom and dad for an answer.

“It can be true,” Robert said. “When you watch the sailboats tomorrow at the race, you may not be able to know for sure which one will be faster. It is not always about the biggest sails or the biggest ship.”

“Boat race! Boat race!” the twins cheered. “Will there be pirate ships at the boat race tomorrow, Dad?” one of them asked. I still could not tell which one was which.

“I don't think so, Jason,” Robert said. “But you will see fast boats and great captains.”

“So, we better go home and go to bed,” Nancy said as she stood up.

She gave me a hug. “You had a long day too,” she told me. “I'm sure you are ready for bed as well.”

I was. After the five of them left for the night, I went to my bedroom and got ready for bed.

I looked at the photo on my dresser one more time. I smiled as I left my windows open to let the breeze in. It had been a long day. It had also been a great day.

Made in the USA
Middletown, DE
27 July 2020

13726161R00033